The Vitiligo Spot Spotter

Story by **Jolene Raison**   Illustrated by **Nikki Naidoo

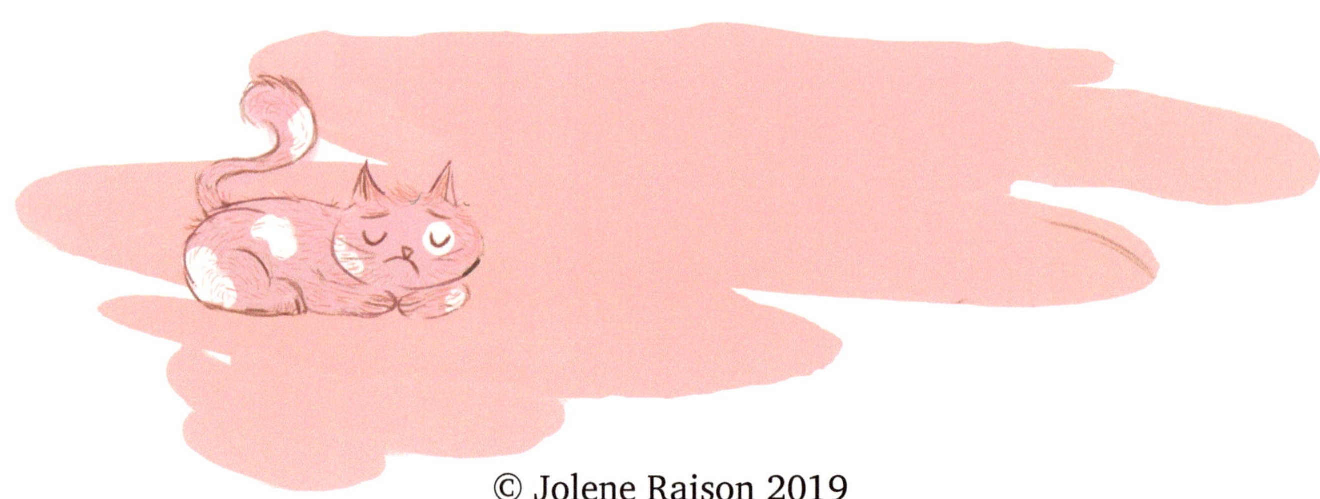

© Jolene Raison 2019

The Vitiligo Spot Spotter

Published by Fishing for Stars Publishing (Pty) Ltd.
P O Box 1274, Glenvista, 2058
jolene@fishingforstars.co.za

ISBN 978-1-7968-6123-5

2 4 6 8 10 9 7 5 3 1

Layout and publication facilitation by Boutique Books
Printed in South Africa by Digital Action

For my son Llewellyn,
spotter of unspottable things.

There's a vitiligo Spot Spotter with a muchness of eyes. A monster of a spotter; a spot spotting spy.

My name is Cinnamon: I'm the one the Spot Spotter spots. I have spots and more spots, but I also have nots. My spots are all white, they're called vitiligo. My nots are the rest of me, where my spots don't go.

Here's the thing about spots: they get lots of
stares. But people look past my nots, like they're
not even there.

Let's say I'm out doing the stuff people do, like
racing my trolley or checking toothpaste tubes,
unpacking the shelf for the ones that I like,
because the best of the best are the ones with the
stripes. (Although toothpaste with spots would
be even better! But no one in the world is near
being that clever.)

So here I am, just doing what it is that I do,
when suddenly I spot them near the frozen food:
a pair of eyes and they're watching me. Then
come more eyes. Two pairs. Now three!

Then it happens: those eyes become more, and
those eyes become more, and in a blink all the
people are gone and I imagine a much-eyed Spot
Spotter right here on the floor. The Spotter does
nothing, it just stands and it stares. But staring *is*
something and its stares make me scared.

It's all eyes on me, and I'm almost in tears. I
wish I were invisible. I wish I weren't here.

So I run.

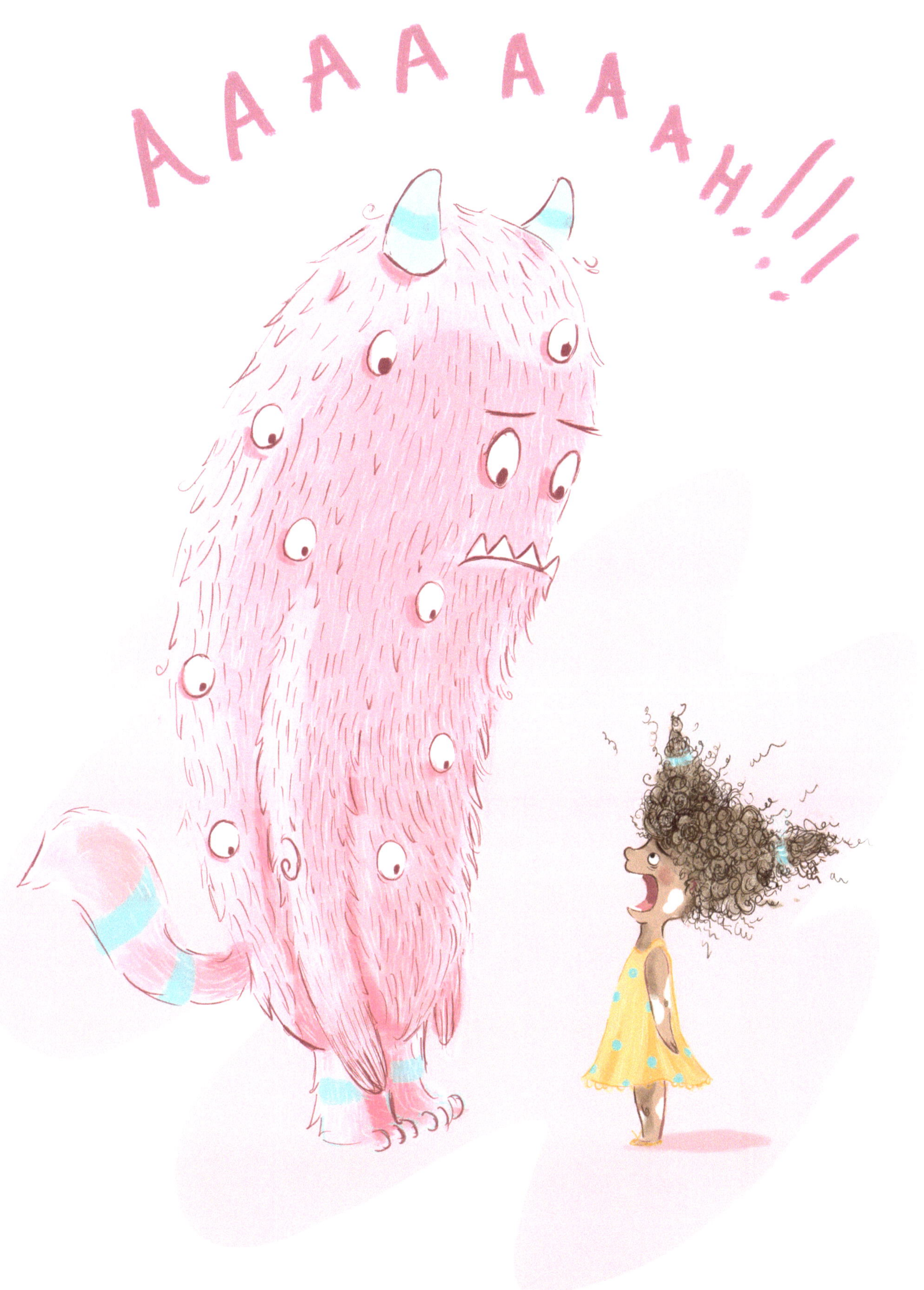
AAAAAAAAAH!!!!

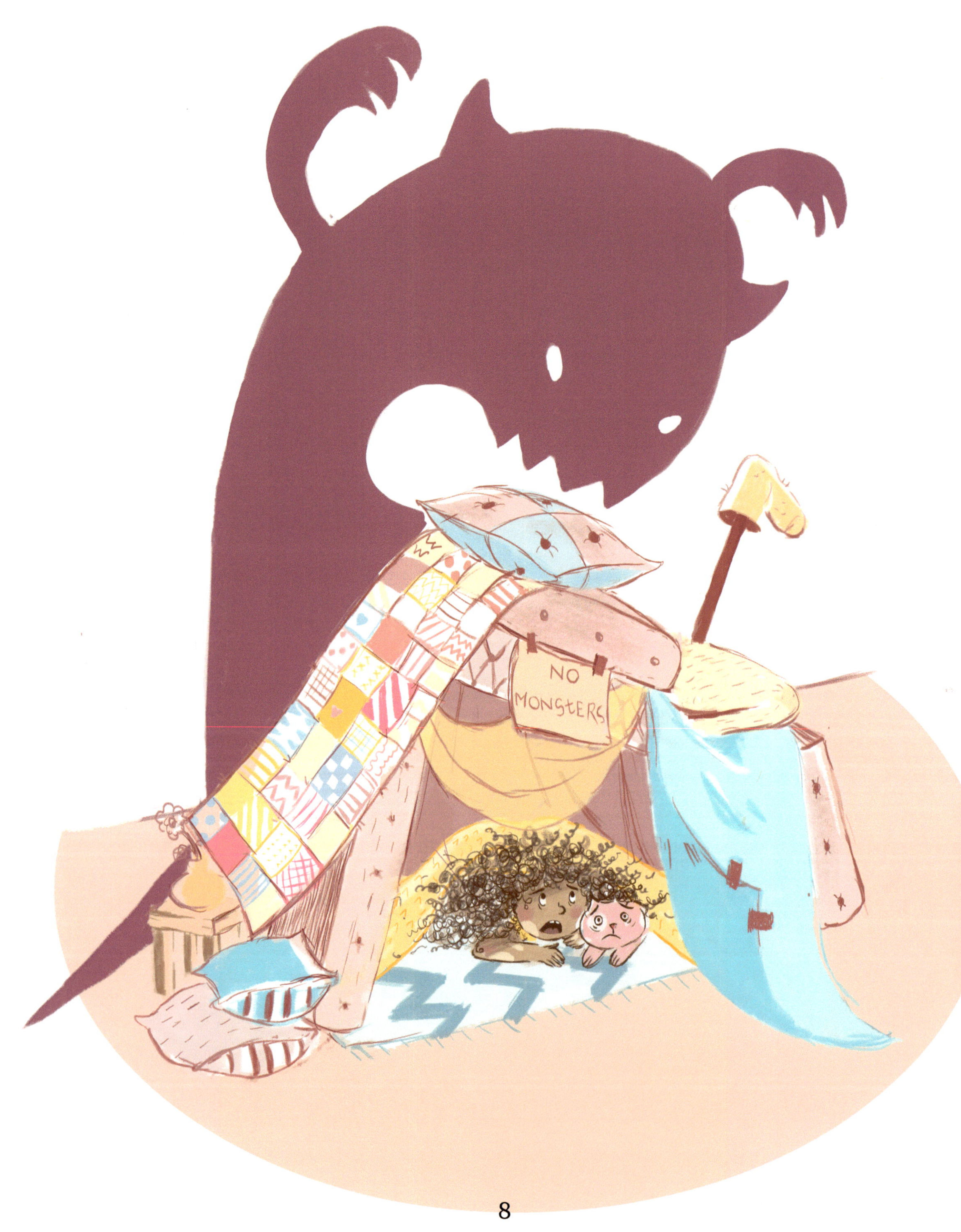

NO
MONSTERS

Can I outrun the Spot Spotter? My legs ache,
but I try. I need to move much faster than the
muchness of eyes. But there are always more
people, there are always more stares – and
where there are people, the Spotter is there.

I run and I run, and I'm finally home. One
door. No eyes. The Spotter is gone.

Or is it?

I sneak a peek through a gap in the curtain.
Could the spotter get in? I cannot be certain. I
check all the corners, check under the couch.
I check all the places a Spotter might crouch.
I look in the mirror. Two eyes, both mine. I
relax. No Spotter. Everything's fine.

No Spot Spotter here, I'm all alone. Our house
is still a stare-free zone! Just to make sure,
I build a fort with Spot Spotter-proof walls.
There aren't any windows – my spots aren't
spottable at all. It has pillows and blankets,
and me in the centre. It has a door that's too
small for Spotters to enter. I can hide here all
day, and all night, safe and sound, and dream
of nots and more nots with no Spotter around.

Unless …

Unless the Spot Spotter got here first. Maybe it's hiding or, even worse, perhaps it snuck in my fort and I didn't see. I imagine the Spot Spotter squashed in here with me. I imagine it's counting every one of my spots. I imagine it's counting an awful lot.

Could we be friends? We might play games. Make shadow puppets. Pretend we've switched brains. I could stick googly eyes all over my tummy, and draw spots on the Spotter – now *that* would be funny.

But the Spotter is scary, it isn't my friend. Quick, switch back! And I'm me again.

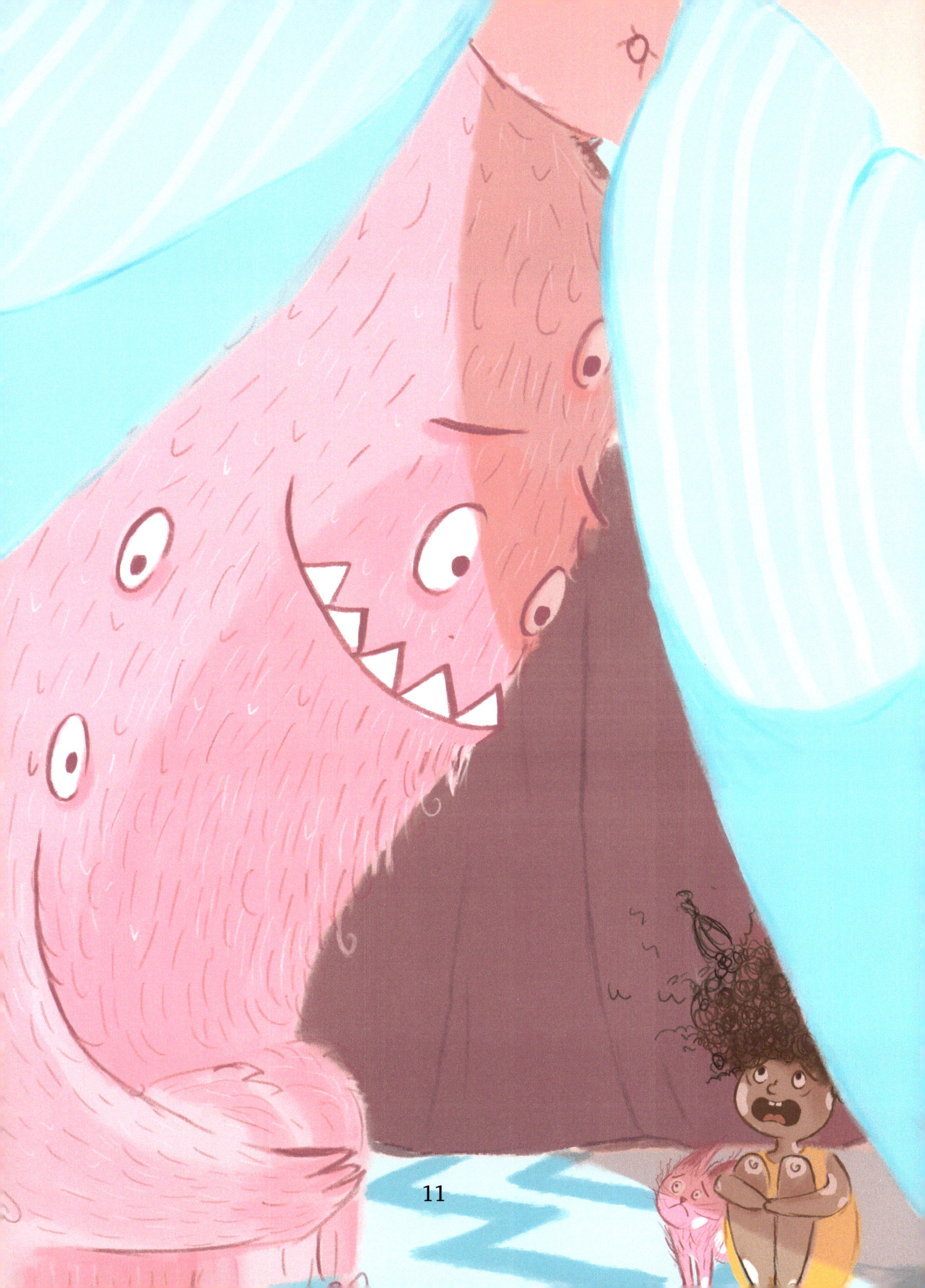

People don't understand about eyes and spot
spotting. They invite me to birthdays and play
dates and shopping.

"We don't see your spots; we think you're so
pretty. You're just as you should be: perfect –
and witty!"

They don't understand – with *their* nots, how
could they? – that their words cannot keep the
Spotter at bay. They've never been scared of a
muchness of eyes, and don't feel too spotty to go
on outside.

I check in the mirror, I scrunch up my eyes,
spotting my spots like I'm in Spotter disguise.
I'm trying to see what a Spot Spotter sees, when
it's spotting my spots and staring at me. I stare
at myself till my eyes start to sting. It's stranger
than strange, this spot spotting thing. I start off
with spots, just the ones that I've got, but then
things get weird: there's a spottery plot. My
spots are growing more spots all over the place,
while my nots start to vanish at a frightening
pace.

Then I blink. And in a second all those new
spots have gone. They were never really there
– there's something strange going on. The odd
thing is that, when I look only for spots, then
that's all I see, and I see a whole lot.

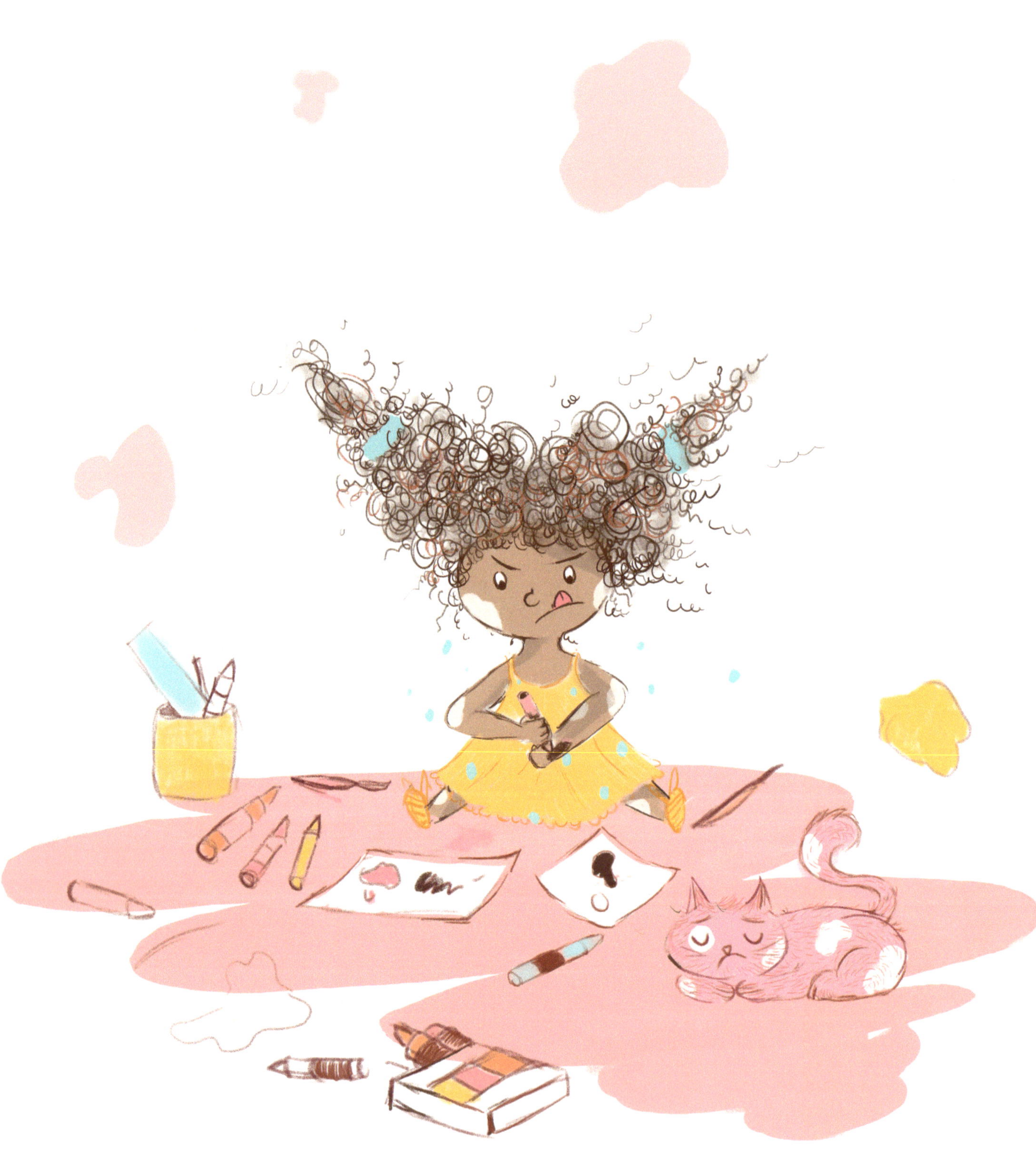

Even if I'm safe here, I can't stay home
forever. I need a plan: something quick;
something clever.

Something like something to cover my spots!
Like wrapping paper … or maybe not. Maybe
crayons, or paint, or pencils or pens. I'll find
the right something and colour them in.

I try every colour, but here is the thing: "skin
colour" can mean a gazillion things. My
colour skin isn't in any box, so now even my
spots are covered in spots. That means double
spots all over me, and twice as many for the
Spotter to see.

If I can't colour *in* my spots, I'll colour *out*
my skin. Then I'll even have spots where
my nots have been, and my spots and my
nots will look exactly the same, and the
Spotter won't bother to spot me again.

I pour a whole bottle of bubbles into the
tub, then I grab a big brush and I scrub and
I scrub. There are so many bubbles, they're
all over the floor. Those bubbles make
bubbles, now they're up to the door. They're
in my eyes, they're in my ears. I scrub and
scrub and hope my nots have disappeared.

But when I peep down through the foam, I
see my nots haven't budged, and my spots
are still spots – they're not even smudged.
In fact, I'm sure there are more than when
I climbed in the tub. Maybe the spots make
more spots the harder you scrub. I know it's
not true, it just seems that way, but there's
no way I'll be spotless or notless today.

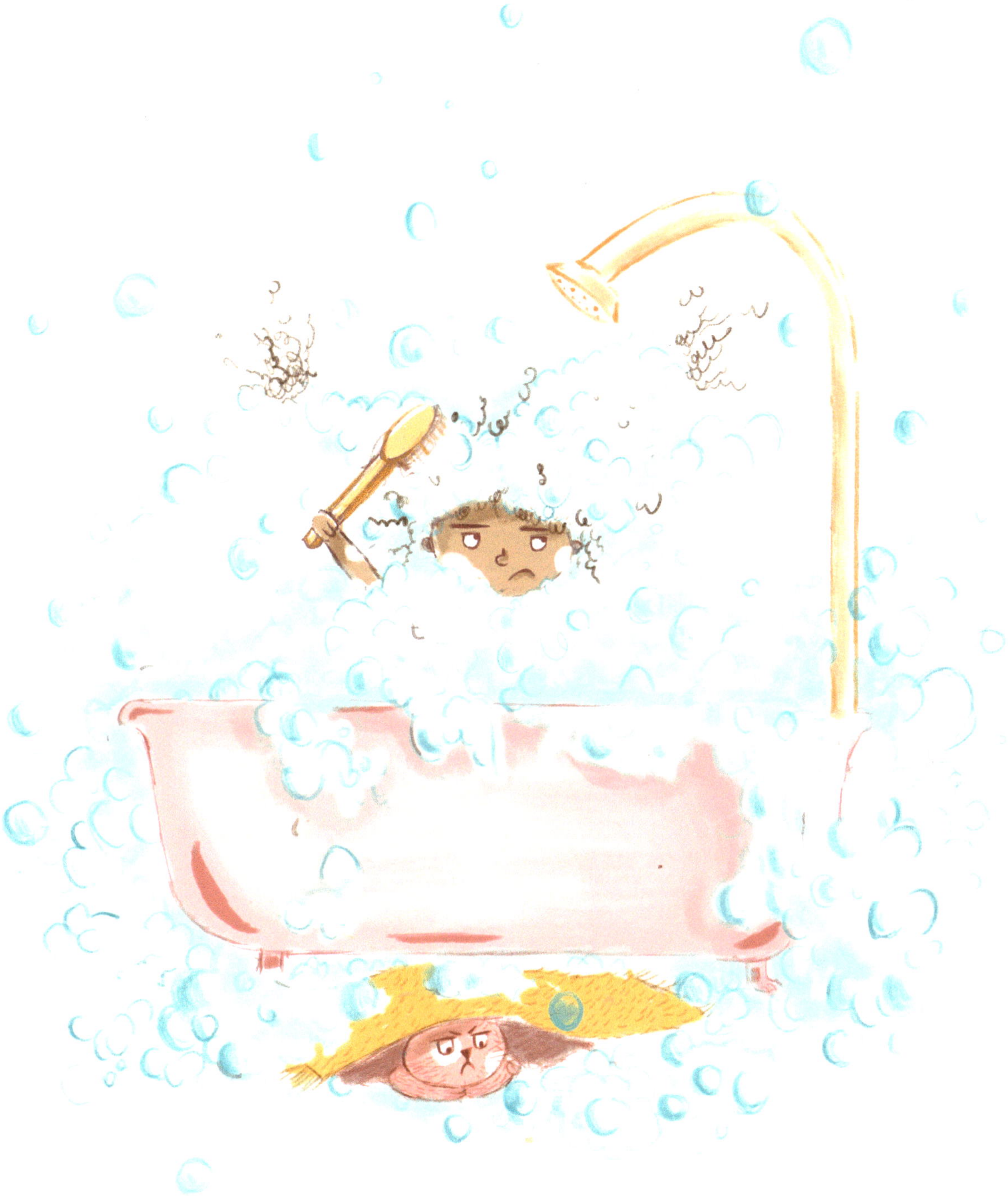

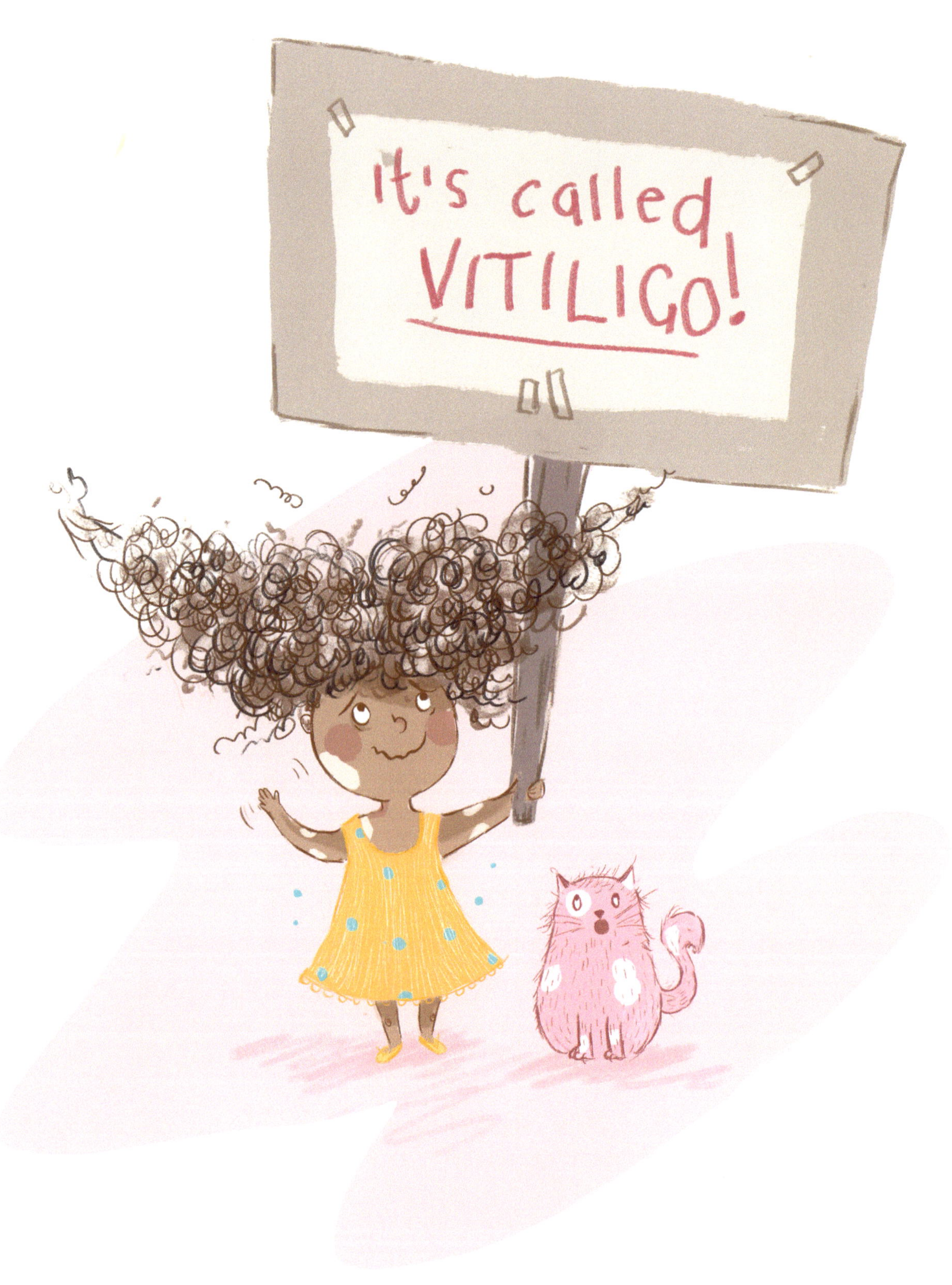

it's called
VITILIGO!

Would the Spotter be friendly if my spots were pretty? Like what if they were green? What if they were glittery? What if they were flower-shaped, what if they glowed at night? What if they were soft and furry? What if they were *striped*? Maybe the problem isn't that I have spots, but that my spots just aren't the right sort.

Or maybe the problem is that Spotters don't know what these spots really are, that they're vitiligo. They're not sure what these spots are about, and that's why they stare, trying to figure it out. I want to yell: "Hey Spotters, don't stare. It's called vitiligo, and I know it's quite rare! No it does not itch or burn or scratch. No you can't catch it if you touch a patch. No I'm not sick, I'm totally fine. It's just that your skin has got more nots than mine."

I've tried to run away, hide away, colour
in and wash away, but it seems my vitiligo
is still here to stay. What I need is a way
to cover myself. I grab the biggest, bulkiest
clothes from the shelf. I cover myself from
my head to my toes: I look like a small
walking pile of clothes.

I'm a bundle of puff, I'm a squishy cloth
bulk, I'm zombie girl, I can hardly walk.
All these clothes are uncomfy, and I can't
really move, but it's this or get spotted – I
just have to choose.

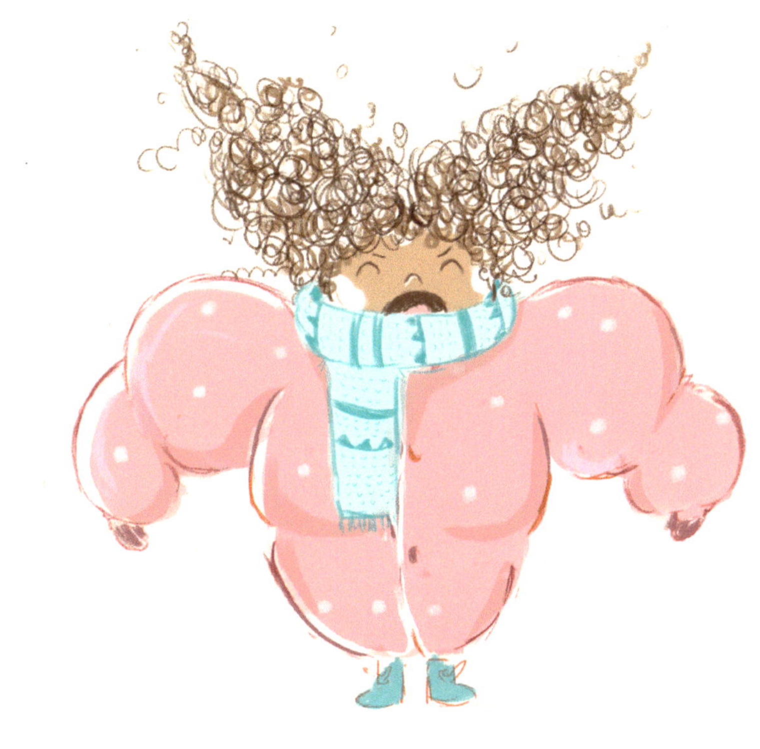

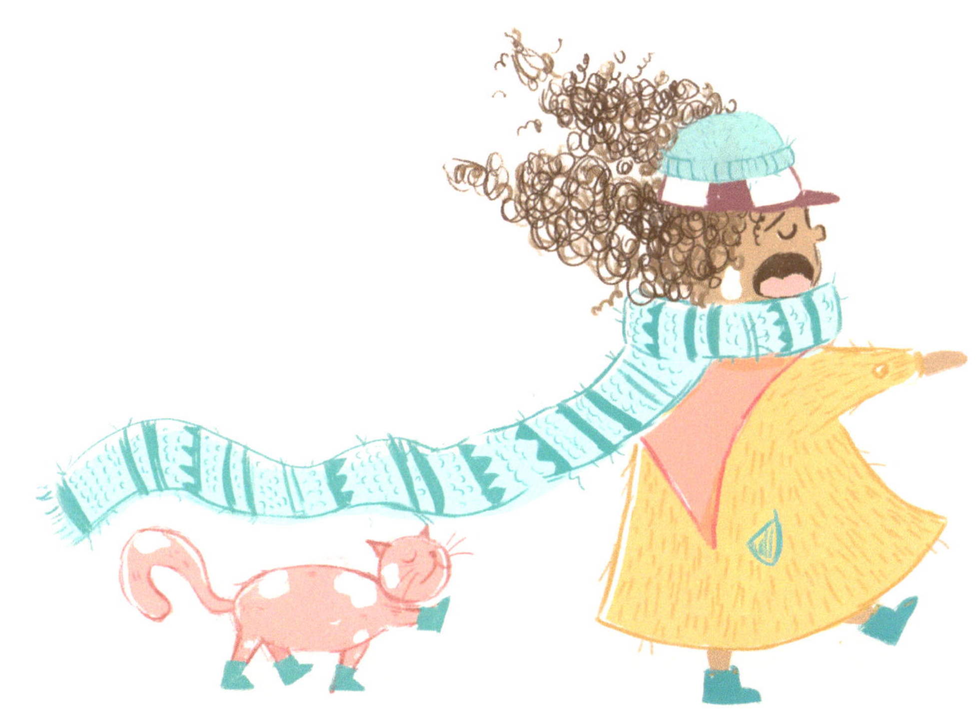

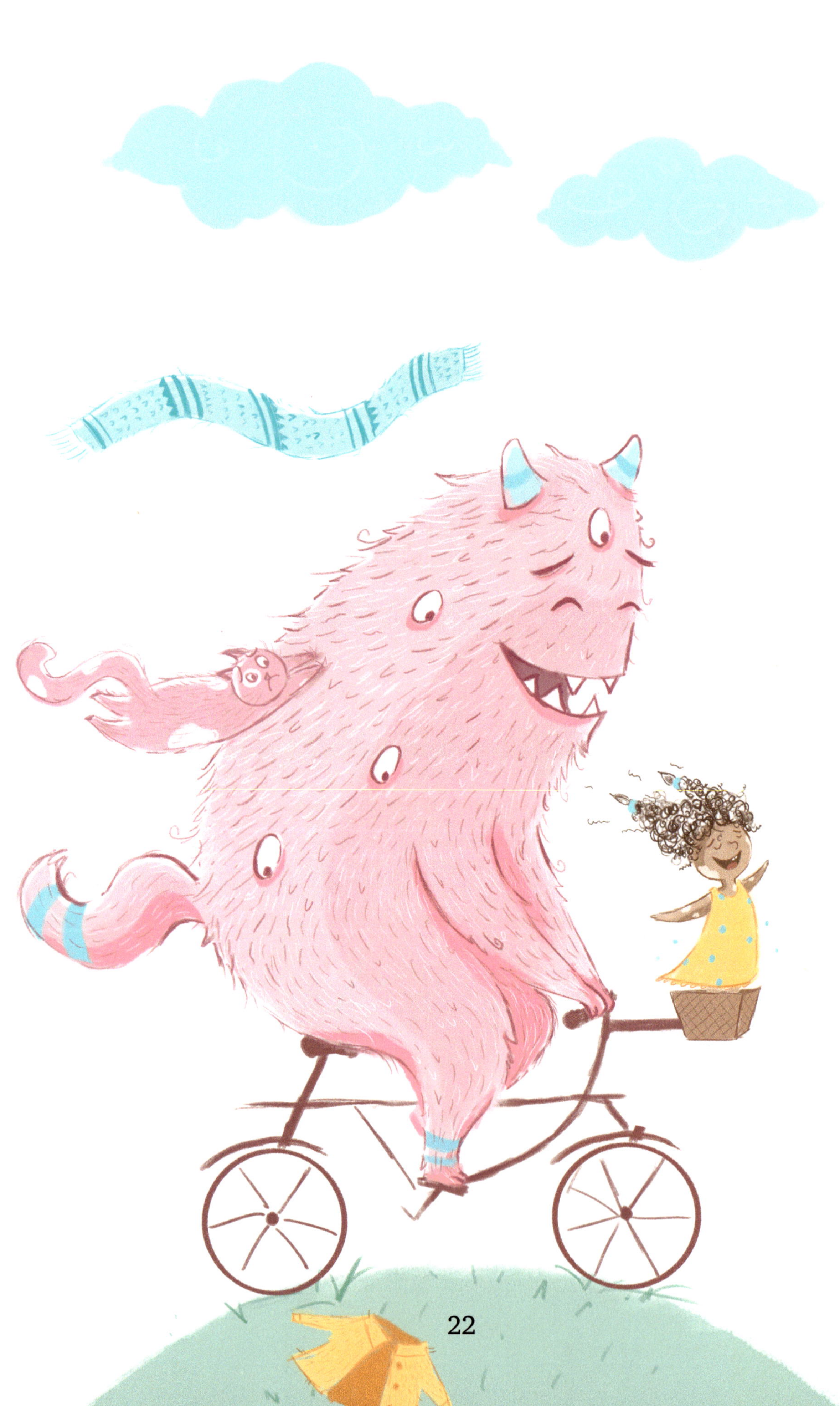

I chose wrong! This is a really bad plan. Can
people melt? I think I am. I start shedding layers,
I'm peeling off clothes. I feel light, I feel happy,
but there's no time to relax. What if the Spotter
is lurking just behind my back? Waiting and
watching and hiding as well? I'm waiting for
Spotter to show itself.

Then it does! But wait, it's not looking at me.
There's someone else here, her spots are like
cherries. She's not running, or covering, or hiding
away. I need to warn her; the Spotter is coming her
way.

"Watch out for the Spotter," I want to shout. But
my spots feel so spotty and the words won't come
out. I want to tell her there's a Spotter and she
needs to scram, but then the Spotter might hear me
and find out where I am.

So I wait.

I watch.

She's just dancing along, this cherry spot girl,
heading for the Spotter, spots blurred as she
twirls. I'm sure she must see it, how can she
not? She keeps going like someone who only
has nots. Now she's whirling and smiling,
arms up in the air, like she's not scared of the
Spotter, like it's not even there.

Then she sees it.

    She stops.

        She does something wild.

She looks the Spotter in all its eyes …

            and she smiles.

The Spotter blinks, it opens its mouth just a
crack, then wider and wider. Now it's smiling
right back!

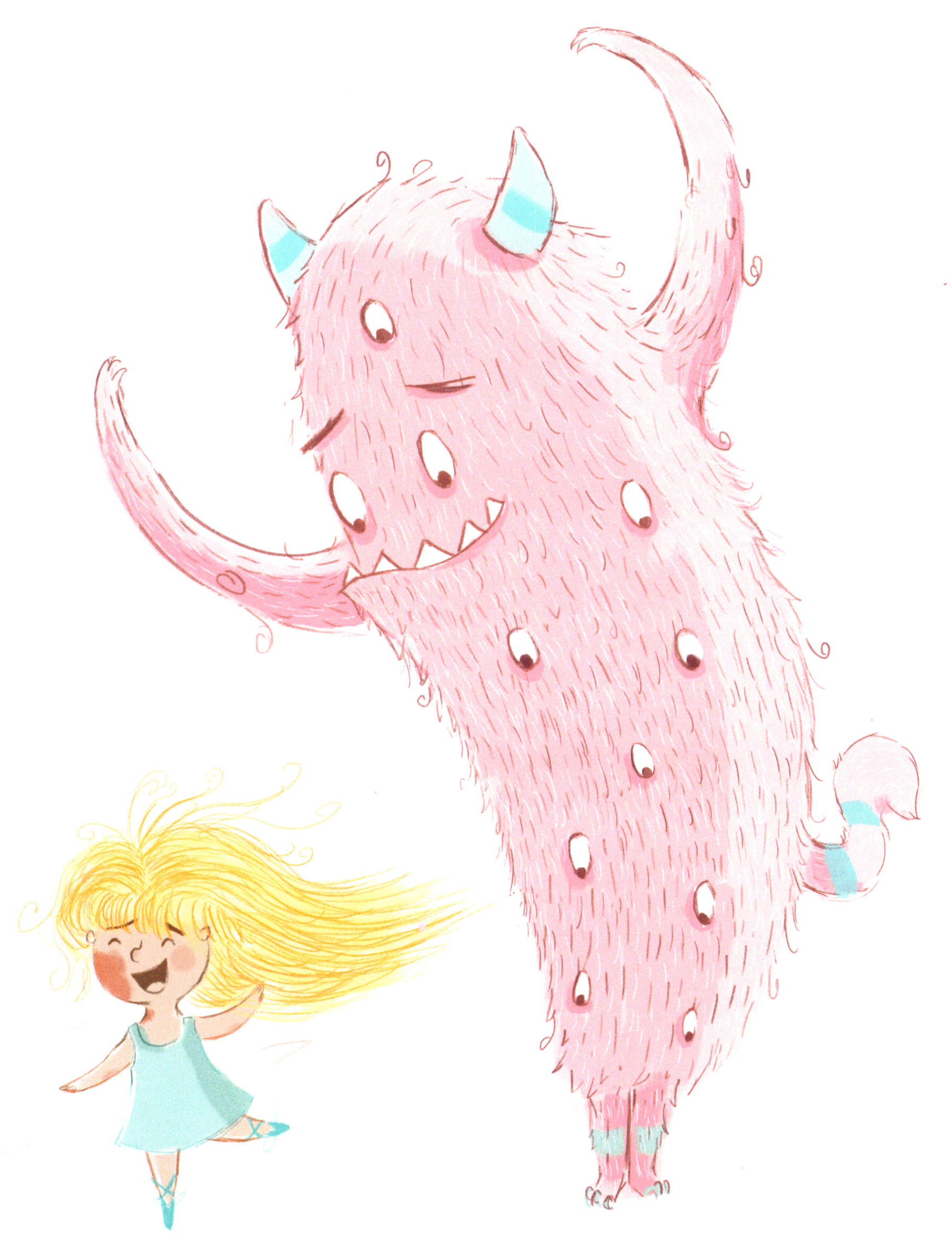

I'm still hiding from the
Spotter, but why isn't
she? Is there some kind
of secret she needs to tell
me?

She says: "The secret

is that Spotters can't do more than stare. And stares are as dangerous as starlight on air. I know that this Spotter has spotted my spots. I know it sees me, but I say so what? *So what!*

"Those eyes might be vicious, or angry or mean. They might be the scariest eyes that I've ever seen. It doesn't really matter what the Spotter can see, the only thing that matters is how *I* see *me*.

"Are my spots something ugly, are they creepy, or odd? Are they some kind of beautiful, something one of a sort? No one can decide if they're bad or okay, these spots are my spots, no one else has a say. I love that I'm the first Spotling whom some people will see. I love that there's no one in the world just like me!"

I think about what she says, I think that it's true. Then I realise: "Hey, today I spot-spotted you. Maybe we're all Spotters sometimes, even me, even you. Maybe we all stare when we see something incredible or new. If a unicorn walked in would we not be amazed? Or a hippo with wings? There's no way I could say that I wouldn't ogle such a radical sight, even though too much staring really isn't alright."

There's a muchness of people, with a muchness of nots, and a muchness of Spotters, but a shortage of spots. Someone spotted like me doesn't come along every day, so all you spot spotting Spotters, please spot spot away!

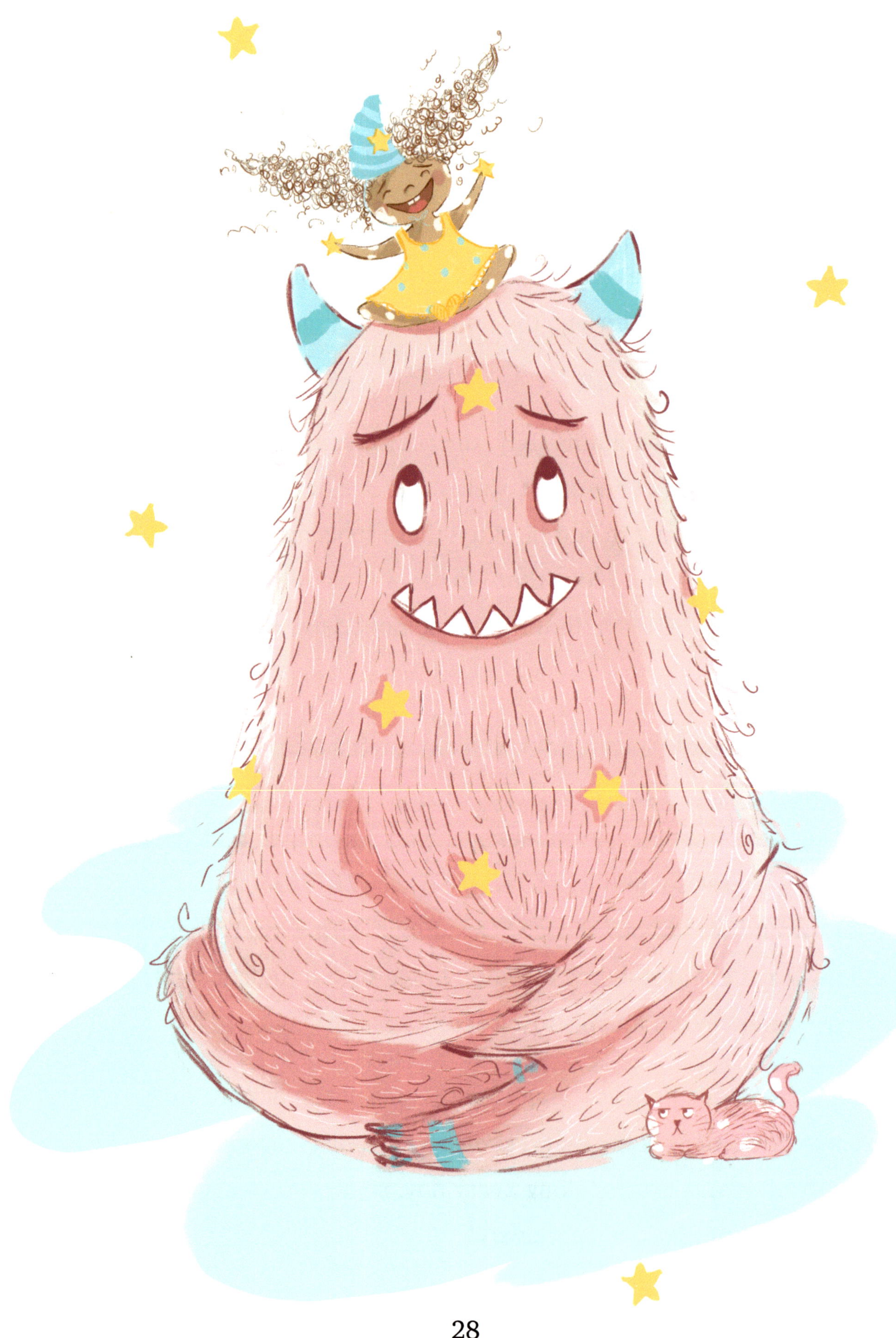

Eyes are just eyes, and a spot's just a spot. It's up to me to decide if they're scary or not.

And the Spotter? The Spotter's not monstrous at all. It could be snuggly or boney or teeny or tall. It could be the friendliest Spot Spotter by far. Instead of eyes, it might have a muchness of stars.

The Spotter is anything that I want it to be, because the one who turns eyes into Spotters is me.

Or I can turn myself into a Spotter of the much-spotted kind, then spot all my own spots, every spot I can find. Because I'm the best Spotter, when it comes to spotting my spots, and I'm learning to love all these spots a whole lot.

The End